# DEDICATION

I dedicate this book to all who feel that hope is lost in losing weight. This book is a perfect guide to have a happier and healthy future just like mine.

# TABLE OF CONTENTS

# Fat Burning Fast: How to Lose Weight Fast and Easy

**Get That Curve – Get that Perfectly Looking Body**

By: Janet Simpson

9781634289719

# PUBLISHERS NOTES

## Disclaimer – Speedy Publishing LLC

This publication is intended to provide helpful and informative material. It is not intended to diagnose, treat, cure, or prevent any health problem or condition, nor is intended to replace the advice of a physician. No action should be taken solely on the contents of this book. Always consult your physician or qualified health-care professional on any matters regarding your health and before adopting any suggestions in this book or drawing inferences from it.

The author and publisher specifically disclaim all responsibility for any liability, loss or risk, personal or otherwise, which is incurred as a consequence, directly or indirectly, from the use or application of any contents of this book.

Any and all product names referenced within this book are the trademarks of their respective owners. None of these owners have sponsored, authorized, endorsed, or approved this book.

Always read all information provided by the manufacturers' product labels before using their products. The author and publisher are not responsible for claims made by manufacturers.

*This book was originally printed before 2014. This is an adapted reprint by Speedy Publishing LLC with newly updated content designed to help readers with much more accurate and timely information and data.*

Speedy Publishing LLC

40 E Main Street, Newark, Delaware, 19711

Contact Us: 1-888-248-4521

Website: http://www.speedypublishing.co

REPRINTED Paperback Edition: ISBN: 9781634289719

Manufactured in the United States of America

# CHAPTER 1- THE TRUTH ABOUT BURNING FATS

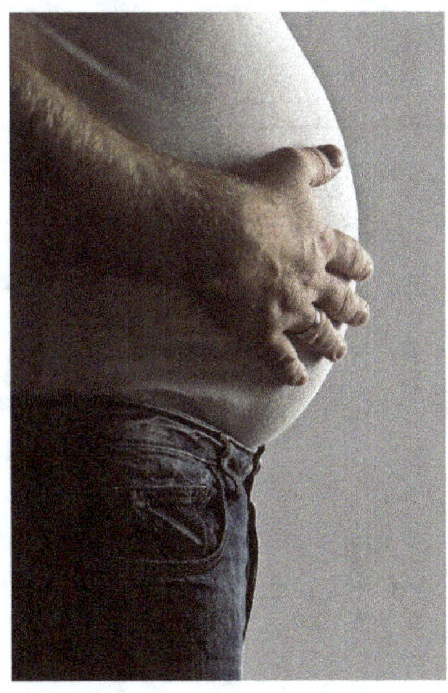

If you're overweight, you are not a bad person. You're simply overweight. But it's important to lose the extra pounds so you'll look good, feel healthier and develop a sense of pride and self-esteem. Once you've lost the fat, you'll need to maintain your weight.

In this booklet, you'll discover how to lose 10 pounds a month – a nice, safe loss of about two or two-and-a-half pounds a week – painlessly. You'll feel satisfied and more energetic than in the past without feeling deprived.

Most Americans pack on those extra pounds by eating the wrong things. Changing these poor eating habits is the key to long-term success. Knowledge – along with the right food – is the key.

When humans lived in caves, they didn't know anything about preserving and storing food. They spent all their waking time and energy hunting and gathering food. When they had it, they gobbled it down fast. Instead of storing food in pantries or cupboards, they stored energy in their bodies in the form of fat to burn during periods when there was little or nothing to eat.

Each year, it was absolutely vital for them to put on a good layer of fat during the warm sprint and summer months. That was the only way they could guarantee their survival during the lean and mean winter months.

And since women bore the young, they needed more energy to sustain themselves and their babies, and that meant they were usually heavier.

Even though we no longer live in caves, we have inherited and maintained this basic mechanism for fat storage from our hunting and gathering ancestors.

Each one of us is born with a certain number of fat cells. How many of these fat cells you possess depend on genetics. If you have a lot of fat cells, maybe your ancestors were the biggest people in the tribe, which was a good thing because they had the best chances of survival.

You can never get rid of fat cells, but – unfortunately – you can add to them. Depending upon what you eat, your body will manufacture new far cells. And like those you were born with, they never go away.

That doesn't mean you're doomed to be fat once you put on extra pounds. It is possible to shrink fat cells. That's what happens when you lose weight. You burn up the fat stored in those big fat cells. Think of them as balloons. Burning off the fat inside them has the same effect as letting the air out of a balloon.

A good weight loss program requires a certain amount of intake restriction – the consumption of fewer calories. You burn off the fat by eating less fat and becoming more active.

To guarantee a lifetime of weight-control success, you have to change the type of foods you eat, so that you ingest less fat and still get the vitamins, minerals, trace elements, protein, fat and carbohydrates your body needs to thrive.

Extremely low-calorie diets may help you shed pounds quickly, but they'll lead to failure in the long run.

That's because humans are genetically protected against starvation. During food shortages, our bodies slow down our metabolisms and burn less energy so we can stay alive.

A part of our brain called the hypothalamus keeps us on an even weight keep by creating a "set point." That's the weight where we feel comfortable. The hypothalamus determines this point based on the level of consumption it's used to. It seeks to keep our weight constant, even if that point is over what it should be.

When we drastically cut back our food intake, the brain thinks the body is starving, and in an effort to preserve life, it slows the metabolism. Soon the pounds stop coming off. Consequently, we grow hungry and uncomfortable and then eat more. And then the diet fails.

How can you compensate for this metabolic slow-down? The answer is that you have to change the nutritional composition of the foods you eat. You will have to cut down on total calories – that's absolutely basic to weight loss. More important, however, is reducing the percentage of total calories you are getting from fat.

That's how you'll avoid starvation panic in your system. At the same time, you reduce the amount of fat in your food, replacing it with safe, low calorie, nutrient-rich plant foods. This will convince your brain that your body is getting all the nutrition it needs.

In fact, you'll be able to eat more food and feel more satisfied while consuming fewer calories and fats.

Plant foods break down slowly in your stomach, making you feel full longer, and they are rich in vitamins, minerals, trace elements, carbohydrates and protein for energy and muscle-building. This allows your body to burn off its excess stored fat.

SPECIAL NOTE BEFORE YOU START

Before You Start.

Before you start ANY new fitness program you need to check with the old' doc first. Really, I know we fitness folks always say this but it's true. Many times we think we can just jump right in but many medications can cause your heart rate to skyrocket. This can put you at risk for all kinds of problems, including heart attack. If you are pregnant or just had your baby please get approval and guidelines from your OB/GYN before introducing exercise. PLEASE, please consult your doctor before starting any exercise program.

# Chapter 2- Fat Burning – The Reason Why You Should Exercise

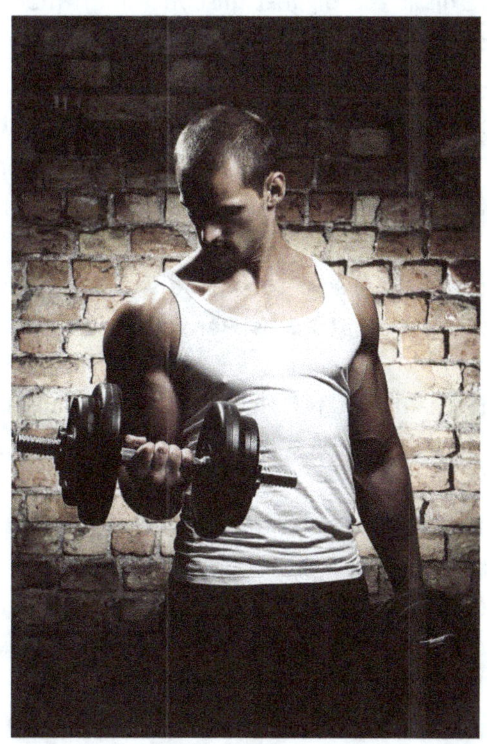

**Why Exercise?**

The main value of exercise is not to burn calories, but to maintain muscle mass (protect the muscle from being burned) and to build muscle mass.

Muscle is a metabolically active tissue. The more muscle you have, the higher your capacity for burning off fat and the faster your weight loss. This because fat is the major source of fuel burned by muscle during sustained aerobic exercise. Also, the more muscle you have, the greater your protection against weight gain.

**Special Note for the Ladies...**

Ladies, I know what you're thinking..."I don't want to bulk up and gain muscle." This is the biggest misconception there is regarding weight-bearing exercise! You will not bulk up from weight training, it's just not genetically going to happen, unless you eat an incredible amount of food, take supplements that support muscle gain, and lift extremely heavy weights. Most women will gain a toned and beautifully sculpted body from weight training.

Another reason to exercise is to expand your energy needs so you pull more fat from your fat stores. Here's how it works:

• Eat a low-fat (I said LOW not Non-Fat) diet and add less fat to the fat stores

• Eat a diet high in fiber. High fiber carbs fill you up so you eat less. Also, think...take it in, get it out!

• Exercising increases your energy needs and increases the amount of fat you withdraw from your fat stores

So, now you understand that you NEED to exercise...but...what do you do to get the most results for your efforts?

**Cardiovascular Exercise:**

Aerobic means "with oxygen". Aerobic exercise is any physical activity done for an extended period of time that forces your cardiovascular system (heart, lungs and blood vessels) to increase the amount of oxygen and blood circulating through your body so you're benefiting even when you are at rest. By increasing your cardiovascular fitness level, you are increasing the rate in which your body burns calories.

**How often do I need to do it?**

30 min/day x 3times weekly is good place to start but for weight loss you could require more depending on metabolism. The first 20 minutes your body burns mostly carbohydrate. After that, the body burns mostly fat. So the longer you exercise aerobically over 20 minutes, the more you will burn.

Having said that, I must also mention that too much cardio or aerobic exercise can work against you. When you do aerobic exercise the body first burns food that you eat, then fat stores and then muscle. If you are doing too much cardio your body will basically eat its own muscle. And the less muscle you have the slower your metabolism will be.

I heard a story by another trainer that really sums this point up. This trainer had a client that was doing very well and staring to really get in shape. She had very balanced weight training and aerobic plan that was helping her reach her weight loss goal. After a while the client was baffled as to why she was no longer losing weight and was not feeling as energetic as before. After her trainer asked a few questions he found that she had increased her cardio to two 60 minute sessions a day! The only people who train this way are seasoned athletes that eat a very specific diet to support such a plan. Her body was basically eating its own muscle, preventing her from losing weight and not to mention really messing up her metabolism. Once she returned to her original plan she continued her weight loss and felt much better.

Moral of this story...more is not always better!

How do I know if I am working out long enough and hard enough?

*Fat Burning Fast: How to Lose Weight Fast and Easy*

For weight loss, duration and intensity are two very important words. Duration refers to how long you are exercising and intensity refers to how hard you are working. When it comes to weight loss, the more aerobic exercise the better (don't go crazy). In my opinion the key is the quality of the time spent doing the exercise that is most important. You will lose more fat walking at various intensities for 30 minutes than running as fast as you can for 10 or at a low intensity for an hour. You may start out walking for 30 minutes but over the next couple of months introduce speed walking or jogging to your sessions. There is something to be said about not letting yourself get in the "cardio rut". Let me tell you a couple of stories to prove my point.

At my gym there is a gal who is the queen on the cardio step machine. Several times a week, you will see her stepping away for at least an hour per workout. She gets on, leans over the arm rails and steps away at the same moderate speed every time. For over two years I watched this gal step…and step…and step. She never changed her routine, intensity or duration and in the process never changed HER SHAPE! She was the same 20-30 pounds overweight as she was the first time I saw her two years prior. I suggested she add intervals to her workout which would put bursts of challenge in her routine and change the type of machine she used at least three times a week. It was going to take her out of the hum drum and into challenge and RESULTS. Sure enough, she started to shed the pounds and make her workouts fun again.

Lessons learned- mix it up and always be challenging yourself!

Let me tell you one more story…

It was Thanksgiving time and mom was preparing the big ham. As she was preparing it the young daughter asked "Mom, why do you cut the end of the ham?" She stopped and thought about it, "Well,

I guess it's because that's the way my mom always did it". "But why?" the daughter replied. "Let's call Grandma and find out". They called Grandma and she said "Well, that's the way my mother always did it". So they called Great-grandma. "Great- Grandma, why did you always cut the end off your ham?" "My pan was too small so I had to cut the end off so it would fit!"

We are creatures of habit. Don't get stuck in the workout rut. If your exercise routine is not getting you results you need, change it up! Don't be a victim of hours on the treadmill at the same slow speed. Throw in a fast minute here and there or increase/decrease the incline every few minutes.

KEEP IT FRESH! Look below for a great interval workout.

**THE ZONE- Target Heart Rate**

To count as aerobic exercise, you need to keep your heart rate in a "target training range" or what some people call "THE ZONE". In order to find out what your "zone" range is you need to calculate your Maximum Heart Rate, or MHR. This is the number of times your heart can contract in one minute.

Max heart rate

220- age = max heart rate (MHR)

Now, multiply your MHR by 65% and 85%. This is your target or training range.

MHR x .65= minimum training heart rate MHR x .85= maximum training heart rate

Ex. 35 year old, MHR = 185 beats per minute Target training range 120-157 beats per minute You want to keep your heart rate in this training range to get the most out of your cardiovascular workouts. Don't waste away, hanging over the machine, doing the same old "hum drum" workout. Get the most out of your precious time!

QUICK TIP: Write this range on your gym water bottle (the plastic re- usable kind). That way you'll never forget what your goal is!

How to measure your heart rate?

The first time you try this I recommend you sit in a chair for a full 2 minutes. Find your pulse using your first two fingers. The best way to do this is to put your two fingers behind your ear and sweep downward to the side of the neck. You can also feel your wrist but it's not as easy to find.

Using a watch or clock count the number of beats for 10 seconds. Multiply that number by 6 and you have your Resting Heart Rate. Use this same technique (don't sit down) while exercising to measure if you are IN THE ZONE.

I wouldn't recommend using the heart rate monitors built into cardiovascular equipment like treadmills and elliptical machines. I'm not sure if I have ever gotten a good reading from one of these things! I would recommend you investing in a heart rate monitor. This will really help you monitor if you are in the ZONE.

**Perceived Exertion**

Another way to measure how hard you are working is measuring your perceived exertion (PE). This is a quick way to rate the quality and intensity of your exercise and stay in tune with your body. When we first start an exercise routine we often feel like we are spent after the first 5 minutes. We need to slowly increase our stamina and therefore will increase our level of perceived exertion. Soon we will be able to exercise for 10 minutes, then 15 and so on. It's about slow, controlled progress.

**BUT HERE'S THE KICKER!**

You have to work! And work HARD! Too many times I see people just strolling along on the treadmill talking to their neighbor. That's not cardiovascular exercise, that's social hour. I can tell they are not in their ZONE. Heck, they aren't even on the playing field!

"But exercise isn't fun and I need to meet my friend so I can take my mind off the fact I'm working out". Sorry to tell ya this but who said exercise is always supposed to be fun! Don't waste your time doing so-so workouts. Wouldn't you like to spend less time in the gym and get more results from your workouts? Then make the most of every second you are there. Quality workouts!

Ok, back to perceived exertion.

PE is on a scale from 1-10. The ZONE is around 7-8. Let me spell it out for you...

Level 1- Totally at rest. Like reading a book.

Level 2- Maybe putting your clothes on.

Level 3- Very easy walking like when you get up to walk to the kitchen.

Level 4- Very light stroll around the block. Normal breathing.

Level 5- This is your warm up pace. You are aware of your breathing but not breathing heavily.

Level 6- Now you're starting to work. You are nice and warmed up.

Level 7- This is your good cardio base level. You are ready, at work, starting to feel slight fatigue and breathing deeply.

Level 8- Shhheww! Now we're working! This is vigorous exercise and you can really feel it burn! Hang in there this is where we make progress!

Level 9- You probably shouldn't stay at this level for long. This is very, very vigorous exercise and you should only experience it for a short time.

Level 10- Woooh nelly! Slow down! You should never be at this level. Are you crazy?

Here's the deal with the PE scale. You are going to want to cheat yourself at first.

Everything is going to feel like a level 9. Let's face it, most of us are out of shape and pushing ourselves to work hard is not at the top of our lists. It will take several sessions to figure out how to manage this scale but you can do it! You really want to master the art of getting in and staying at level 7-8.

This is your ZONE! If you want to change your body into a fat burning, calorie eating machine you need to get in and stay in this ZONE. Remember...your level 7-8 is very different than your friend's level 7-8. You cannot compare PE scales!

# CHAPTER 3- THE EFFECTIVE CARDIO FOR FAST FAT BURNING

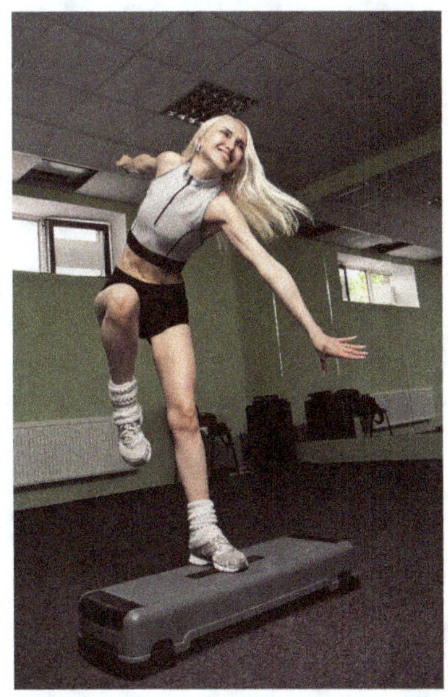

The one you actually will do! The best of exercise to decrease fat stores is steady, rhythmic, and continuous, i.e. aerobic exercise. There are some forms of cardio that are more effective than others. To break it down to the ridiculous...here's a list from best cardio burn to activities that should be a supplement to your regular exercise. You want to stay at the top of the list:

**SUPER CHOICES**

- Power walking

- Lap Swimming (continuous) Jogging

- Aerobic dance/ class

- Stair climbing (actual climbing or simulation machine not step machine)

- Elliptical machine

## GREAT CHOICES

- Stair stepping

- Stationary Bike (the upright one) Recumbent bike (the low seat one) Rowing machine

- Spinning

- Cross country ski machine or Arc trainer

## GOOD CHOICES

- Roller blades

- Outdoor biking- recreational Sports

- Dancing, gardening, house cleaning

## INTENSITY

Now that we know what exercises to do, now we need to talk about how to do them. Intensity is extremely important when it comes to getting the most calorie and fat burn during exercise. Besides don't you want to get the most bang for your effort...I know I do.

Tips:

Don't just get on the treadmill and walk at the same moderate pace the whole time. Remember your training heart rate range!!!! Try this routine to mix thing up a bit:

**30 Minute Interval Workout**

Level is your perceived exertion scale of 1-10. 1=easiest and 10=hardest To make the intensity level higher you can increase speed, resistance or incline.

Warm-up 5 minutes Minute

TIPS TO REMEMBER:

• 30 minutes on the treadmill or bike too hard for you right now? Try 10 minutes walking, 10 minutes biking and 10 minutes on an elliptical glider. MIX IT UP! But don't quit!

• Do the talk test. Can you carry on a complete conversation with your buddy on the machine next to you? You're probably not hitting your target zone. On the other hand, if you can't catch your breath enough to say "call 911" you are most likely at the upper end of your range and need to bring it down a bit.

In addition to weight control, aerobic exercise:

• Improves cardiovascular fitness

• Lowers blood pressure

• Relieves insomnia

• Strengthens, tones, and shapes

• Shown to reduce risk of some cancers, such as breast cancer

**Running 101**

So you want to start a running or jogging program. According to the American Council on Exercise you need to start with the following:

1. Check with your doctor first.

2. Purchase a pair of quality running shoes. Don't just go to the discount shoe mart and get the $20 special. You will save yourself a lot of pain and suffering if you start off with a shoe that meets the needs of "your" foot type. I would recommend going to an athletic shoe specialty store and have them fit you for the right pair of shoes.

3. Pick a place. Find a place to run that is safe and well lit. I would recommend that you rotate 2-3 locations because you never want to run at the same time and place each session. Predators look for victims who have patterns in their schedules. Also, when picking a place to run chose asphalt or dirt over concrete surfaces.

**Good Form is Essential**

• Keep your head level, avoid bouncing and lean forward slightly

  from the ankles.

• Keep your shoulders down and relaxed.

• Strike the ground first with your heel, then roll to the ball of the

  foot, pushing off the toes.

Don't go gangbusters all at once. Pace yourself by starting off with 30-45 minutes 3 times a week with days off in between. Stay within 50-85% of your max heart rate.

If you prefer to have a plan ACE recommends the following beginners program.

| Week | Minutes | Intensity |
|---|---|---|
| 1 | 20 | Walk |
| 2 | 22 | Walk |
| 3 | 22 | alternate 30-60 sec jog then 5 min walk |
| 4 | 24 | " |
| 5 | 24 | alternate 30-60 sec jog then 4 min walk |
| 6 | 26 | " |
| 7 | 26 | alternate 30-60 sec jog then 3 min walk |
| 8 | 28 | " |
| 9 | 28 | alternate 30-60 sec jog then 2 min walk |
| 10 | 30 | " |
| 11 | 30 | jog 2 minutes then walk 1 minute |
| 12+ | 30 | keep this progression |

Remember running isn't for everyone. If you don't like it, don't do it. Walking is great also.

**MY BIG FAT EXCUSE CORNER**

I have heard it all before my friends. Sometimes we will find every reason to justify why we shouldn't exercise when we should be looking for solutions that will help us to fit it in instead. Here are a few…see if they strike a nerve.

1.      I don't have time to exercise 30 minutes/ 3 x week!

Let's talk time management, priorities and attitude! If you want to make positive changes in your life and improve your health YOU WILL FIND TIME! Go to bed earlier so you can get up before work, take the kids and bike or walk after work or dinner, tape your favorite evening TV shows and take the family to the gym instead. Adding exercise to your routine will actually help you sleep better and have more energy. You're not going to be more tired by exercising! You will actually have more energy to get things done, can you imagine?

Ask yourself these questions:

Do I understand why I need to exercise?

Am I willing to do what is necessary to fit this exercise into my schedule? What activities or exercise do I enjoy most?

What equipment do I have? Can I get?

Can I go to the mall and walk? At lunch? After work? Can I ride my bike or walk to work?

Can I get up early and walk or do a video workout? Can I involve my family in my quest for better health?

Am I ready to make the changes to my lifestyle that I know I need in order to achieve better health?

"You will never "find" time for anything. If you want time you must make it."

**Charles Buxton**

2. I can't exercise, I have a bad ankle, foot, back...brain).

Do you really? Or did you 5 years ago? Absolutely, consult with your doctor before starting any exercise routine BUT don't just assume the injury or problem you had years ago means you can't exercise today. I have clients that had serious back problems improve significantly from a gradual and safe exercise routine. As they got stronger, so did their back. They ended up improving their quality of life significantly. Don't let yourself fall into the "I CAN'T" rut.

3. I don't like exercise. I can just lose weight without it!

You can lose weight if you don't exercise, but it will be slower and less permanent than if you add aerobic exercise. By not exercising you will lose muscle, your fat-burning tissue. This will slow down your weight loss and make it more difficult to maintain. Plus, exercise isn't all about the weight loss! It's good for your lungs, heart, blood pressure, cholesterol, sleep, mood....I can go on and on. It's good for you and makes you feel good and strong.

Now, let's move on to the next MUST HAVE element of your exercise plan...strength training...

# CHAPTER 4- FAT BURNING – ENDURE PAIN, GAIN STRENGTH

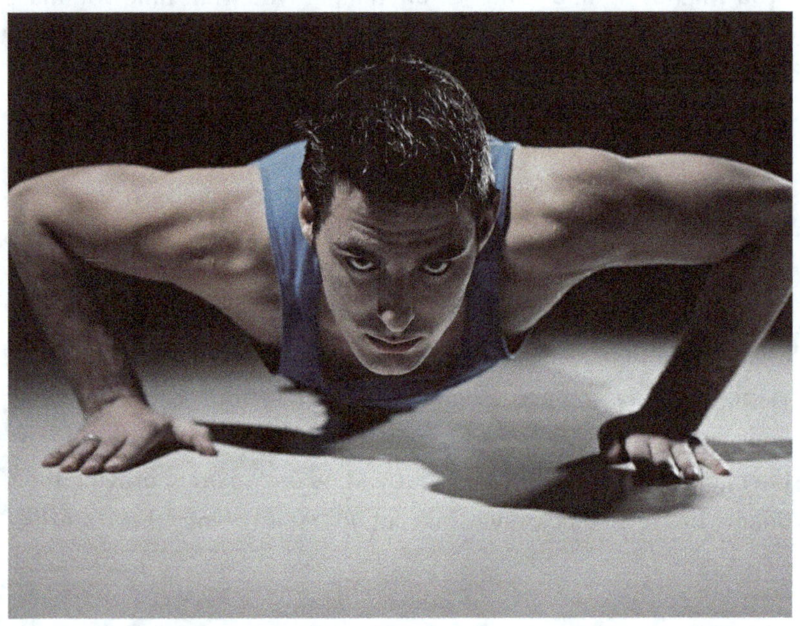

Strength training is anaerobic exercise. Or exercise done in short, intense bursts that works your body without requiring much oxygen. So, when you lift weights you are trying to reshape your muscles from flab to tone and fab. Basically, you working the muscle against some form of resistance in order to break it down and rebuild it stronger and leaner.

When it comes to weight training you need to know a couple of basic terms. Repetition- the number of times you lift a weight or complete an exercise Set- a group of repetitions of the same exercise performed without stopping.

I do cardio all the time. Do I really need to train with weights?

Absolutely! Weight training strengthens your body and allows you to perform better during cardio sessions, which will help you burn more fat. Muscles are calorie burners and weight controllers so build them up and be a real loser…weight loser that is!

How often do I need to strength train?

According to the American Council on Exercise, 2-3 times a week is plenty. But for those we need to lose a significant amount of weight or those who desire BIG results a bit more quickly…3-4 may necessary. Consult with a certified trainer to start off slowly and to find out how to develop the right routine for you and your goals.

How much weight and how many reps should I do?

I recommend you start your lifting routine with 12-15 reps per set. There are many techniques that incorporate heavier weights at lower reps but stick to the basics right now. Start with a low weight that you know you can lift.

Continue increasing the weight until you reach a weight that makes you feel fatigued after 10-12 reps. Keep a lifting log and chart your progress. As you get stronger you will need to increase your weight. Always be asking yourself "did I feel the burn on those last few reps?" If not, increase your weight.

Do I have to lift using just machines or hand weights?

There are many different machines and gadgets you can use in your strength training routine. Here are just a few:

• Gym type machines- Nautilus, Cybex, Hammer Strength, Life

• Exercise bands or tubing

• Hand weights, bar bells and medicine balls

• Cable machines and towers

I find the most effective strength training routines are done right at home with a set of hand weights and maybe an exercise band. If you have a routine you can do at home you won't have any excuse! If you have a gym membership you can have a member of the fitness staff give you an orientation on the equipment or just schedule a personal training session.

This will help you feel much more comfortable in the gym and make sure you understand proper form on the machines.

How do I know what exercises to do?

There are a few rules to remember when weight training:

1. Warm-up for at least 5-10 minutes at a low intensity. This will increase blood flow and reduce chance of injury.

2. Make sure you are doing exercises that get all of the main muscle groups, not focusing only on legs or only on arms. You must have balance to avoid injury and build a strong and lean body all around.

A trainer can help you develop the right set of exercises but to start keep it simple. Focus on:

• Upper Body Chest  Back Biceps Triceps Shoulders

• Lower Body Quadriceps Hamstrings Calves Glutes

• Core Abs

• Low Back

3. Use proper form. I don't know how many times I have seen someone at the gym lifting weights that are entirely too heavy for them. They are swinging around every which way trying to lift it and completely disregarding form. They would gain so much more out of the movement if they would lower their weight and maintain proper form.

4. Breathe! Geeeze, stop holding your breath already! Holding your breath during exercise can put unnecessary pressure on your heart and increase blood pressure. Just remember to exhale on the exertion and inhale on the release.

5. Start off with low weights. One of the biggest mistakes I see with those new to weight training is that they lift too heavy, too soon. There's nothing like muscles so sore you can't move for a week to send you back to the couch and TV.

6. Get your rest. Your body must have rest in order for your muscles to repair and recover. Lack of rest will only slow your progress and weaken your immune system.

"But I do crunches every day and still have a big belly!" There is no such thing as spot reduction! AND YOU CAN QUOTE ME ON THAT! If your goal is to get your belly under control you must have a clean diet and most importantly DO YOUR CARDIO! You need to burn that layer of fat off that is in front of your abs. Eat right, do cardio and weight train and you will see your belly go from Pillsbury Dough Boy to The Rock in due time.

Things to remember when working the abdominals or "CORE":

Core means torso stabilization and involves your tummy and back working together. The muscles that make up this region are the:

- Rectus abdominis

- External obliques

- Internal Obliques

- Transverse Abdominis

I tell you this because if you just do traditional old hands behind the head crunches you are missing many other muscles in the core area. You MUST mix it up...upper abs, lower abs, obliques (side abs).

- A Quick Note About The Abdominals and Core:
- Never pull on the neck
- When holding hands behind head keep elbows angled outward and not crowding the head.
- Don't jerk or go too fast. Take your time and get the most out of each repetition.
- Perform the movement slowly and controlled.

Now, cardio revs your system, burns fat and calories and is incredibly good for your lungs and heart. Strength training builds lean muscle tissue, helping the fat burn process and makes you look darn good! There's a couple of more forms of exercise that I won't lump into either cardio or strength...they are kind of cross-breeds that combine stretch, relaxation and strength all together. I think everyone should at least try these and add them once or twice a week to their routine.

**Yoga**

Yoga can be a four letter word to some people. I have suggested it to many of my clients only to get an eye roll or "you gotta be crazy woman".

Truth is, most people fear it because they only know it as the pretzel-like positions made fun of on TV sitcoms. There are many forms of yoga, look for gentle styles such as Kripalu, Viniyoga, or Integral Yoga. Bikram, Ashtanga, and Power Yoga are generally too vigorous for beginners and inflexible people. If you are weary of the eastern philosophy and meditative practices of some yoga classes not to worry. You can find many yoga type fitness classes offered at local gyms and YMCA's that are philosophy-free but still very calming and true to the movements.

Many of my clients ask me about the "hot yoga" classes that are all the rage right now. I decided to try one out before I would give my opinion. Wow, what a workout! However, I would not recommend it for everyone. Most hot yoga studios will screen you before you sign up but if you are on ANY kind of heart or blood pressure medication I would speak with your physician first.

# CHAPTER 5- IMPORTANT NOTES THAT YOU NEED TO KNOW ON FAT BURNING

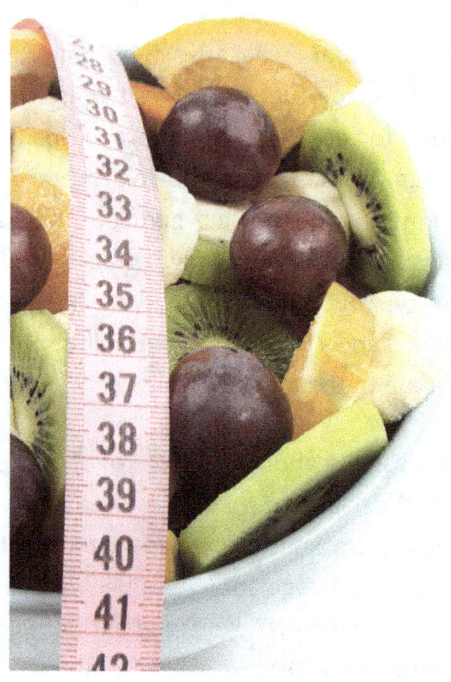

• Diet Food Is Not Healthy & They Do Not Work (Did you already know that Aspartame has been diagnosed to cause symptoms of cancer? There are a number of chemicals that are used in this diet or "health" food that are actually very toxic to our bodies. If you look at what ingredients diet food has, you'd be surprised at the amount of different chemicals within that are very unnatural to our bodies. Nobody knows what will happen to your body after consuming diet food for a prolonged period)

• Weight Loss Business Is A Repeat Business: If you get thin, they would be out of business. That's why you hear about more and more unbelievable stuff being put out for you to buy. Most diets don't work because they are not supposed to work. The diet industry involves HUGE amounts of money and it doesn't make sense (from a business point of view) for them to get you thin. It's a license to print money at the expense of your health.

• Eating Different Food In Certain Patterns Can Easily Make You Lose Weight: One of the most effective ways to lose weight is a method that makes your body's metabolic levels run high and your body burn fat in a natural way. Any external gimmick is bound to result in automatic failure (such as pills, potions). Why use gimmicks when the answer can be found within your own body?

• Working Out Is Not An Effective Way To Burn Fat (A workout has only a 20% effect on your weight loss journey. If you eat the right way, it's going to have up to an 80% positive effect on your body weight)

• By Keeping Your Metabolic Activity High You Can Lose Weight Without Any Extra Diet Food, Weight Loss Pills Or Any Other Gimmicks (that have little or no effect but empty your hard earned money from your wallet)

Real Reasons Why You Are NOT Losing Weight

• You Believe That "Diet Food" Or "Health Food" Or Other Light Products Make You Thin: If you find yourself searching for the next great light meal or some diet food when you are grocery shopping or always asking for a diet coke, then you are facing a problem that many others are experiencing. You are trying to lose weight with the wrong products. All gimmicks such as "light food" or "diet food" are not going to get you anywhere besides spending your hard earned money. These things are only there to get you into a vicious cycle of gaining weight and even health problems (because these "health foods" tend to have quite a lot of chemicals in them and some artificial sweeteners have even been reported to be dangerous to consume(Aspartame to name one) )

- You Are Consuming Too Much High-Carb Food: Trying to eat all kinds of salads in hope of losing weight does not work. During the day you might eat bread, rice and other high-carbohydrate meals. It's been researched that carbohydrates trigger the brain to crave even more of it. This ends up causing a cycle which leads to eating becoming harder to control. As a result, you might be taking all kinds of snacks during the day. By engaging a high protein (and low-carb) diet you are not only going to feel hungry less often but it turns your body into a fat-burning machine (because your body needs a lot of energy to digest that meat).

- You Don't Have a Clear Goal: Weight loss as any other goal you might have should be clearly stated. "I want to lose XX pounds in XX days". For more about setting goals, look at the chapter concerning this matter more closely

- You're Counting Calories And Not Concentrating On Positive Results: This has been discussed many times over, but if you focus on how many calories you should take and so on, you are not concentrating on anything else such as the positive results you should have from your dieting. Your thoughts become negative, leading to negative results. Find out what type of diet or lifestyles are beneficial to weight loss and follow them. It's as simple as that. For the calorie counters: It doesn't matter if you count your calories or not, because your body will adjust to the diet very quickly. In other words: if you eat fewer calories, your body will spend fewer calories. It's simple and stupid.

# Chapter 6- Effective Methods to Fast Fat Burning

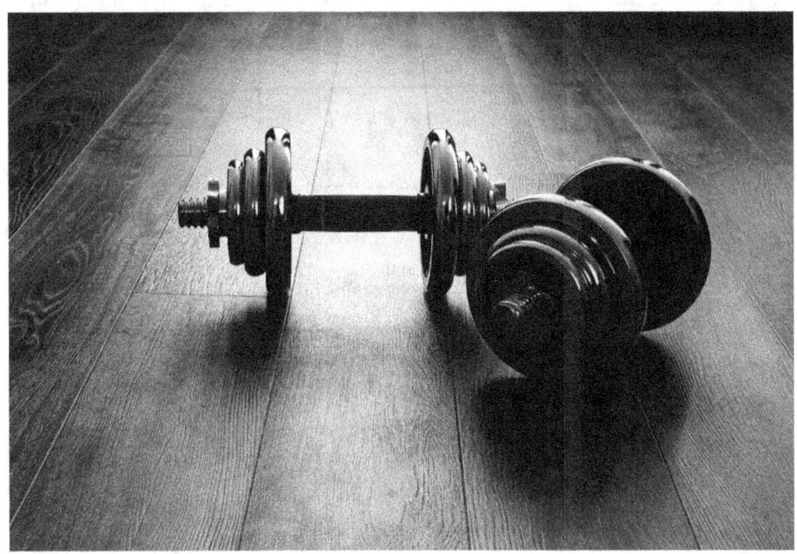

**1. "Metabolism Booster" Method**

This method is about a conservative weight loss method. It's not a rapid way, but it's excellent if you really want lose weight steadily and for the long term. You can also keep your ideal weight once you've used some of the quicker methods below. But as we all know that if you want to keep your weight from fluctuating, then you should be aware that most of the quick diets yo-yo your pounds back in no-time. To avoid this, you should watch what you eat as well as the quantity.

1. Eat at least 6 or 7 times a day

2. Never eat too much. You should always stop right before you are full

3. Drink lots of water on a daily basis (Remember the 8x8 rule: Eight 8-ounce glasses of water per day that is around 1.9 liters)

4. Don't do heavy exercises, but regular walks of at least 30 minutes every day (6x a week)

5. Pure, organic food without any conservative chemicals (Many readymade "TV-dinners" contains many toxic chemicals)

6. Try eating as much as protein every meal as you can (but still remember rule #2)

7. Avoid carbohydrate products such as spaghetti, rice, potatoes, bread but instead eat fresh vegetables

This is not as strict as a low-carb diet, but more of a lifestyle you should be following because high-carbohydrate meals tend to make people fat. Forget about salad-only meals because it doesn't give you the protein you need. Turkey, Sea bass and other types of "white" meat are good for this purpose.

Always try to replace the high-carb ingredients with vegetables whenever possible.

## 2. "Kill The Carbs" Method

Low-carbohydrate diets have been around for a long time and there is still some controversy about whether it's safe or not.

Before you start this diet, you must understand that this might be rather taxing on your body so be sure to consult your physician before undergoing it. People with kidney disorders should not try this. The same precautions apply to pregnant women as well as people with diabetes.

The basics of a low-carbohydrate diet are about eating protein rich food so that your body doesn't use carbohydrates as the main source of energy, but rather your own body fat.

There are different phases in this lifestyle (or you can take it as a diet as well):

1. Induction: Your carbohydrate intake must be less than 20 grams for the first 14 days. Following that, your body will enter a state of ketosis. This means that your body will burn its own fat because it's accustomed to get that energy from your carbohydrate intake. When that is not available it will use the body fat to get energy instead. This is an extremely effective way of burning fat.

2. Then you should be gradually increasing the carbohydrate intake by about 5 grams a day. You are going to reach a state where the total amount of carbohydrates is around 30-90 grams per day. Once you spot an increase in your body weight, you should go 5 grams back. What amounts to 5 grams then? A handful of peanuts, one cup of strawberries, etc. Know your food and be careful about it.

Check your local library for a list of what amount of carbohydrate a particular food has.

You should also get some vitamins because you might initially feel drained as the state of ketosis prohibits you from eating large amounts of fresh vegetables. Exercising should also be on your daily menu, but not a hard workout. Instead, walking or some other light activity will be far more effective for this cause. Once you stop this diet, you should be VERY careful about how much and what you eat because if you don't watch out, the pounds can come back very quickly.

## 3. "Shift Those Friggin' Calories" Method

A calorie shifting is something people have had tremendous success with. It's about giving your brain the thought that your body has gotten a good healthy sized meal with many calories. The result of this is that it will start burning more calories than you've taken in. However, this is by no means about counting any calories. And because you are eating in certain patterns, your body does not get used to any single pattern and adjusts for it by lowering your metabolism. Instead, your metabolism is kept high at all times, which results in effective fat burning capabilities.

The best part of this diet is that you are eating from all the food fields that your body needs; vegetables, fruits, meat, etc - so it's very natural and going to get that fat burning at a high rate. Nevertheless, you need to be strict about the amount you are eating. You should not exceed a certain amount of a particular food type.

This method also brings about quite some variety and you can even choose from the various food types once you find something attractive and tasty. Despite that, you need to first have a balanced diet that your body is accustomed to. Hence, in order for this to work, you should have a normal diet comprising normal food like a regular breakfast, healthy lunches and a proper dinner. This is the foundation which works as a springboard for your calories shifting program.

Day 1: High Calories (+400 cal)

Day 2: High Calories (+200 cal)

Day 3: Low Calories (-500 cal)

Day 4: High Calories (+100 cal)

Day 5: Low Calories (-400 cal)

And So On (Variation is the key – your metabolism thinks it's going to get a basic amount of energy, but then it gets less – You lose weight)

You should not be eating more or less than 4 times a day (every 2, 5 – 3 hours).

You must be aware that there are certain food types you should be eating others you should abstain from.

Get a good book listing calorie values of different food and make a list items that you're about to eat. Then simply make a 10-day plan shifting calories daily. You should make that list once and then never look back on your calories. If you think only about how many calories you've eaten, you become insane just because you have to watch and read everything all the time. Just make a list of your food and then just follow your plan. Don't over-complicate matters.

**Why Going To The Gym Is Only Good For Firming Up Your Body And Not Effective For Quick Weight Loss**

Let's face the facts: If you really want to lose weight quickly, then going to the gym is not the answer, because it has been researched that your body does not effectively burn fat from a hard workout, but instead from what you eat.

Sure, working out is healthy and should be endorsed but it has little to nothing to do with quick weight loss.

*Fat Burning Fast: How to Lose Weight Fast and Easy*

Instead of killing yourself at gym, what you should do is have a healthy walk for at least 30 minutes a day. Only 30 minutes daily can (and certainly will) result in better health, increased energy and more weight loss (when connected with a proper diet).

By having this type of walks daily, you will get into better shape and your weight will definitely go down.

Quick instructions:

1. Tempo should not be too quick

2. Walking and talking should be possible the same time

3. You should be ready for a quick walk without any preparation and equipment

4.      The longer the better, 45 or 60 minutes will not harm you, quite the contrary

**Positive Affirmation Great Contributes**

You should always set goals when losing weight. If you don't set your goals, then it's very possible that your whole dieting plan might not go the way you imagine it.

List the following:

1. What is your current situation right now? List all your eating habits, food preferences, everything that could affect your weight loss. Working out, etc

2. What is the reason you want to lose weight? This could be an upcoming event, summer, or even for a certain special someone. List the single BIGGEST reason you can think of.

3. What are the benefits you get from your weight loss? List AS MANY as you can. It can be health, better energy, admired by partner, etc. This should be your main motivator.

4. Your Goal. "I want to lose XX lbs of weight in XX days" - Write this in bold and make it really sink in. I would personally say that putting more than 10 lbs per 2 weeks is not realistic, especially if this is your first attempt at a goal like this. Be realistic. You must write "I want" not "I wish"

Write everything down and look at that paper every day. Put it into a place where you can see it. Once you see it every day, you will constantly be reminded of WHY you do this and what the benefits are.

BE PERSISTENT ONCE YOU TAKE ACTION BECAUSE IT'S NOT GOING TO BE EASY STEPPING OUT OF YOUR COMFORT ZONE. You must definitely want to lose weight.

If you see yourself making excuses rather than STARTING a diet that is effective, you should think about why you don't really want to lose weight. You must be able to step out of your comfort zone and JUST DO IT!

# Chapter 7- Keep it Low to Make Fat Burning Effective

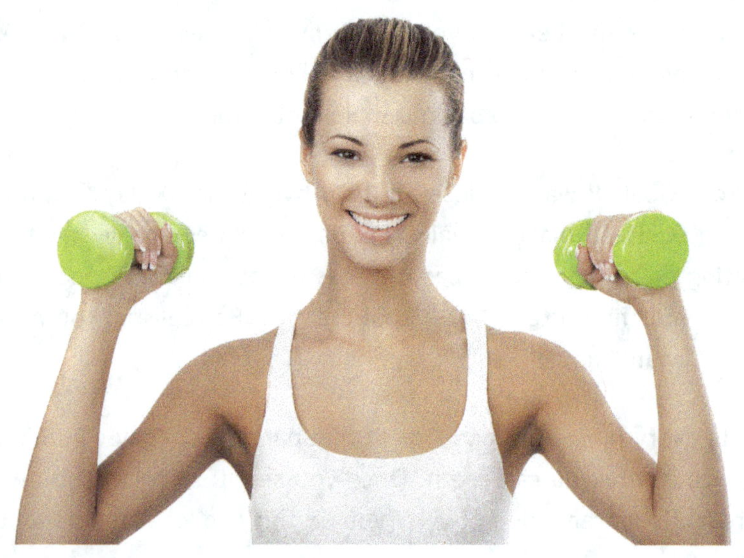

Myth: you'll burn off more fat if you work out at lower intensities versus higher intensities during cardiovascular activities.

Reality: all right, this is technically true, but you have to look at the total picture to comprehend why this would really work against you if you're attempting to slim down.

If you're working out at a low intensity, say 50-60% of your maximum pulse, we're probably safe to say that more than one-half of the calories you're burning off come from fat (let's suppose 60%), and the remainder (approximately 40%) come from sugar, or carbs, in your bloodstream and in your muscles. Bottom line, you burn a greater share of fat at this intensity level than carbs.)

In case you aren't acquainted with intensity based on pulse, 50-60% of your maximum pulse is an easy pace, something you likely could sustain for a long time, perhaps hours.

When you're exercising at greater intensities (suppose 70%-80%), we're safe to state that most individuals are burning off a higher percentage of carbs than fat. Now, simply from this info alone, it may be easy for individuals to believe they're burning fatter at the lower intensities, correct?

The percentages are sure enough greater at the lower intensities. So you may see why so many individuals thought this was the better way to burn fat.

Well, let's have a closer look at what is truly occurring. Let's suppose you've a choice to work out at lower or higher intensity, and let's presume two additional things: 1) among your fitness goals is to drop off body fat and 2) you've a particular amount of time to do your aerobic training; for the sake of this illustration, let's suppose you only have a half-hour. Let's utilize a real world example. We'll call her Joan. One day, Joan works out at 60% (low intensity) of her maximum pulse on the treadmill and she burns off 150 calories. If we may safely say she's burning about 60% of her calories from fat, then she burned off about 90 of those calories from her fat stores. And, if the other 40% of calories burned off came from carbs, then she burned 60 calories from carbs.

The following day, Joan does a higher intensity (80% max pulse) exercise on the treadmill (you have to compare utilizing the same mode of exercise), and she burns 310 calories in a half-hour. If 40% of those calories hailed from fat and 60% from carbs, then she burned 124 calories of fat, and that leaves 186 from carbs.

So, while Joan burned a greater portion of calories from fat with a lower intensity exercise (60% vs. 40%), her absolute value of calories burned off of fat was better in the higher intensity exercise (124 fat calories) versus the lower intensity exercise (90 fat calories). Do you understand why this is a myth and where it may have come from?

Let me make this truly simple. In terms of dropping off body fat, it is not the absolute number of fat calories that counts as much as the absolute number of calories altogether. To exercise off one pound of body fat you have to burn an additional 3500 calories, whether you accomplish it with low intensity or high intensity. I'm sure you are able to see that if you're a busy individual, it pays to get fitter so that you may burn more calories in less time.

However, there's a crucial point about fat burning and intensity level. It has to do with "time to fatigue". Fatigue may impact how many calories you burn. Let me explain.

When Joan is walking at 111 bpm, or 60% of her maximum pulse, if she had the time, she could continue going and going, for a really long time without getting tired. But when she's moving on the treadmill at 148 bpm (80% of her maximum pulse), after a half-hour, she's dog-tired! She's very little energy left. She wasn't fit enough to do that.

Let me explain how fat and carbs get into play here. When you're chiefly utilizing fat as an energy source, as in the case of Joan exercising at 111 bpm, a lower intensity for her, your body may continue to manufacture energy without running out of it. Put differently, it will take a while to tire. However, when you work out at greater intensities, you utilize a bigger percentage of carbs. As the percentage of carbs increases, the sooner you'll tire.

Why is this crucial? I want you to fully comprehend how fat and carbs play a role in exercise and weight loss. Firstly, fats and carbs are equally crucial as energy sources when it comes to exercise.

Secondly, one supplies slow, long-term energy (fat) and the other supplies quick and powerful energy (carbs). Intensity of work out impacts which energy source will prevail over the other.

Thirdly, your intensity level ought to be based on your goals. If your goal is to burn off as many calories as possible in the quickest amount of time, you need to exercise closer to the top end of your capacity.

If your goal is to exercise for a lengthy time period and optimize the number of calories you burn, you'll need to pace yourself. If you merely wish the health benefits, you need to accumulate half-hour a day of activity, which may include exercise and general activity.

Note that the better way to avoid burn out but sustain high levels of fitness and calorie burn is to use interval training, interchanging short bursts of higher intensity training with longer periods of lower intensity training.

Finally, don't forget that the first goal of any exercise program is consistency. It's crucial to begin at your current fitness level and slowly progress in little increments.

# Chapter 8- Fat Burning While Sleeping

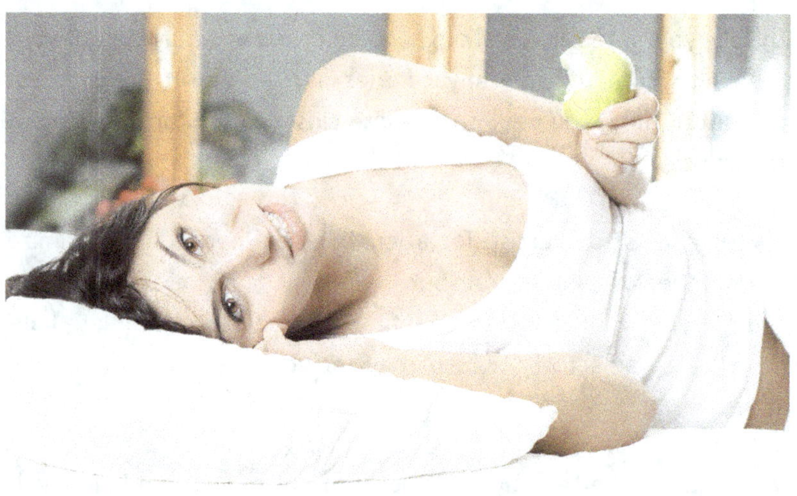

You already burn up fat while you catch some Z's, without any trick pill or potion. You don't have to fess up, but how many times have you tested some burn-fat-while-sleeping merchandise? It's understandable why you'd do so. It appears simple, it doesn't require any time, and it appears to work for famous persons! As we talked about earlier, at lower levels of activity, or no activity in the least, we're predominantly utilizing fat as our fuel. As a matter of fact, you're burning fat right now while reading this book (you are able to thank me later...). When you sleep, you're likewise burning off fat.

As a matter of fact, researchers have now discovered a link between the length of sleep you get every night and your weight. In one field of study, over 68,000 ladies were asked to describe how much sleep they got as a rule every night. For sixteen years, the research workers tracked the participants' weight. Final results demonstrate that ladies who got 5 to 6 hours of sleep a night gained more weight than those who slept at least 7 hours every night. One researcher stated, "Short rest duration is an independent predictor of later weight gain and incident obesity".

In a different study, both gentlemen and ladies were queried about their rest patterns. They discovered that those who got 7 to 8 hours a night were thinner than those who slept 5 to 6 hours. They likewise discovered that those who got less sleep likewise had lower levels of leptin, a hormone that plays a role in body fat and appetite. It's believed that these individuals might be leptin resistant, and consequently they don't get the appetite-suppressing result from it.

Now, what if you could you burn off more fat while you rest? You may accomplish this by increasing your metabolism. I understand, easier said than done. It calls for work and patience for this to occur. And, if you slim down, your metabolism really drops as your body has less weight to carry around. All the same, there's a way around this. The way to supercharge metabolism is to increase the total of muscle you have on your body. Now don't panic about becoming bulky or looking like those ladies in the muscle building magazines. They get that way through a lot of hours daily at the gym, a really stern diet, and occasionally a little help from a few banned substances. Most ladies could never look like that, even the ones who wish to.

So, to step-up the amount of muscle you have, you have to integrate strength training. The crucial thing to remember is that for each pound of muscle you have on your body, you'll burn around thirty-five to fifty extra calories a day. This number is deliberated inside the exercise physiology world, but each pound of fat you have will burn off only two calories a day. So whatever number of calories it truly is that muscle burns, it will be entirely more than fat. If you're active and utilizing your muscles (during exercise, for instance) you'll burn off even more calories per pound during the activity.

And so the bottom line here is that in order to burn fatter while you sleep and all throughout the day, you have to strength train to better muscle and your metabolism. Next time you discover a commercial for the new metabolism increaser, spend your cash on some dumbbells alternatively.

**When to Exercise**

Is morning is the better time of day to work out to burn body fat.

Well if you aren't a morning person, then morning isn't the best time to work out!

As you are able to imagine, there has been far-reaching research on this subject. A few of the research studies recommend that we work out in the mid-afternoon for the most beneficial results. There are a lot of reasons for this, but one is that this time of day falls under the correct time based on our innate biorhythms.

So that's great, let's all go exercise at 2pm each day! Perhaps these researchers may take the time to work out at 2pm, but most individuals I know can't. They have occupations, or they have to fit in workouts around their children's agenda, and a lot of additional reasons.

I don't know who began the idea that it's better to exercise in the morning. Wherever it came from, I've seen this recommendation a lot of times. I read once that you'll burn fatter in the morning as long as you don't consume anything before exercising. There's no way that's going to work for me! For one thing, I have to eat something before I exercise; it's simply the way I am. Second, I'm not a morning individual. It takes a few hours for me to maneuver at full power. If I work out at this time, I really end up burning less calories and I don't get my pulse to the intensity I wish. I'm not burning off much fat this way! It's a big waste of time.

By trial and error, I've found that 10am is the most beneficial time for me to work out. Luckily, I have the sort of schedule that I may fit it in at that time. If I worked regular hours at an office, I'd exercise at lunch, as that was the closest to my ideal time.

So one matter to think about when attempting to ascertain the most beneficial time for you to work out is what time of day you feel you're finest. A different way is to determine what time of day you'll really follow through with your work out.

A lot of individuals discover they need to exercise first thing in the morning as if they hold off, the whole day will go by and they'll find excuses for not working out. Others like to work out when they get home to work off tension from their jobs.

I recently met someone who had trouble sticking with a workout schedule. This had been an issue for years; she would exercise for about 3 weeks, then it would go to pieces. She liked to work out after work as she has a nerve-racking job. This worked for a while as she was motivated and she had a coach to hold her accountable.

Finally, she found more and more reasons to skip her exercises. She decided to attempt working out in the morning prior to leaving for work. After a few weeks of getting used to it, she discovered that the exercise truly helped her by giving her the energy she required to deal with her job. She ultimately found a schedule that would work for her.

And so the bottom line is if you limit yourself to working out when the so-called authorities say you ought to, you'll find yet another barrier to taking control of your personal health. Let your body and your life-style dictate the best time for you. Don't fret about burning fat better at one time or another.

**Eating and Exercising**

Should you or shouldn't you eat right before/after exercise?

Unless you're an athlete, there are no rules!

This isn't precisely about burning off fat. But if you're attempting to slim down, I'm certain you have wondered about this. I've heard that you ought to eat following exercise to replace glucose and glycogen supplies. I've likewise been told not to eat following exercise in order to heighten calorie burn. To be truthful, I don't know what you ought to do or shouldn't do. I truly don't think anybody does.

Here is just a little sample of advice from a lot of respected authors and health associations:

• Avoid arduous exercise for at least 2 hours following eating a

  meal.

• Wait approximately twenty minutes before eating following

  exercise.

- Eat something light 30 minutes prior to exercising in the morning. Make sure to eat inside 2 hours after to restore fuel to your muscles.

- Work out in the morning on an empty stomach.

- Consume a low fat, complex-carbohydrate meal or snack one to four hours prior to exercise.

- Eat .45 gm of carbs per pound of bodyweight one hour prior to exercise.

Like I stated, I truly don't think anybody knows for certain. In my judgment and experience, everybody is different, you have to experiment with when, and what you ought to eat before and/or following exercise. If you eat prior to exercise and you feel sick to your stomach or sluggish, you likely should cut down on the amount or not eat at all. If you feel dizzy or weak, you might have to eat more or eat closer to working out. If you're hungry following exercise, that's a great indication that you ought to eat! In all cases, make sure to eat when you're hungry and stop when you're full.

The concept of intuitive eating works here, too. If you feed your body established on its physical needs and demands, you'll eventually return to your natural weight. Bottom line, you'll have to experiment with when you eat and the sorts of food you eat to ascertain what is best for your body.

# CHAPTER 9- FAST FAT BURNING FOODS

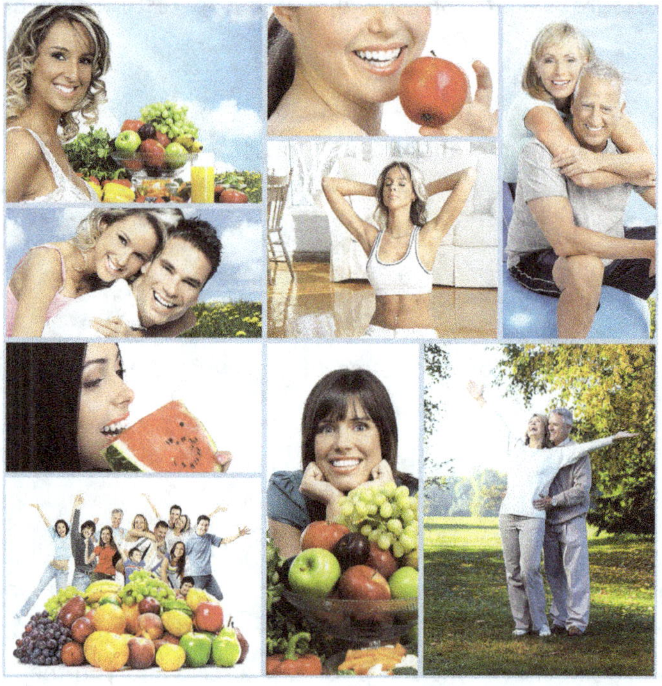

Each one of the following foods is clinically proven to promote weight loss. These foods go a step beyond simply adding no fat to your system – they possess special properties that add zip to your system and help your body melt away unhealthy pounds. These incredible foods can suppress your appetite for junk food and keep your body running smoothly with clean fuel and efficient energy.

You can include these foods in any sensible weight-loss plan. They give your body the extra metabolic kick that it needs to shave off weight quickly.

A sensible weight loss plan calls for no fewer than 1,200 calories per day. But Dr. Charles Klein recommends consuming more than that, if you can believe it – 1,500 to 1,800 calories per day. He says you will still lose weight quite effectively at that intake level without endangering your health.

Hunger is satisfied more completely by filling the stomach. Ounce for ounce, the foods listed below accomplish that better than any others. At the same time, they're rich in nutrients and possess special fat-melting talents.

## Apples

These marvels of nature deserve their reputation for keeping the doctor away when you eat one a day. And now, it seems, they can help you melt the fat away, too.

First of all, they elevate your blood glucose (sugar) levels in a safe, gentle manner and keep them up longer than most foods. The practical effect of this is to leave you feeling satisfied longer, say researchers.

Secondly, they're one of the richest sources of soluble fiber in the supermarket. This type of fiber prevents hunger pangs by guarding against dangerous swings or drops in your blood sugar level, says Dr. James Anderson of the University of Kentucky's School of Medicine.

An average size apple provides only 81 calories and has no sodium, saturated fat or cholesterol. You'll also get the added health benefits of lowering the level of cholesterol already in your blood as well as lowering your blood pressure.

## Whole Grain Bread

You needn't dread bread. It's the butter, margarine or cream cheese you put on it that's fattening, not the bread itself. We'll say this as often as needed – fat is fattening. If you don't believe that, ponder this – a gram of carbohydrate has four calories, a gram of protein four, and a gram of fat nine. So which of these is really fattening?

Bread, a natural source of fiber and complex carbohydrates, is okay for dieting. Norwegian scientist Dr. Bjarne Jacobsen found that people who eat less than two slices of bread daily weigh about 11 pounds more that those who eat a lot of bread.

Studies at Michigan State University show some bread actually reduce the appetite. Researchers compared white bread to dark, high-fiber bread and found that students who ate 12 slices a day of the dark, high-fiber bread felt less hunger on a daily basis and lost five pounds in two months. Others who ate white bread were hungrier, ate more fattening foods and lost no weight during this time.

So the key is eating dark, rich, high-fiber breads such as pumpernickel, whole wheat, mixed grain, oatmeal and others. The average slice of whole grain bread contains only 60 to 70 calories, is rich in complex carbohydrates – the best, steadiest fuel you can give your body – and delivers surprising amount of protein.

**Coffee**

Easy does it is the password here. We've all heard about potential dangers of caffeine – including anxiety and insomnia – so moderation is the key.

The caffeine in coffee can speed up the metabolism. In nutritional circles, it's known as a metabolic enhancer, according to Dr. Judith Stern of the University of California at Davis.

This makes sense, since caffeine is a stimulant. Studies show it can help you burn more calories than normal, perhaps up to 10 percent more. For safety's sake, it's best to limit your intake to a single cup in the morning and one in the afternoon. Add only skim milk to tit and try doing without sugar – many people learn to love it that way.

**Grapefruit**

There's good reason for this traditional diet food to be a regular part of your diet. It helps dissolve fat and cholesterol, according to Dr. James Cerd of the University of Florida. An average sized grapefruit has 74 calories, delivers a whopping 15 grams of pectin (the special fiber linked to lowering cholesterol and fat), is high in vitamin C and potassium and is free of fat and sodium.

It's rich in natural galacturonic acid, which adds to its potency as a fat and cholesterol fighter. The additional benefit here is assistance in the battle against atherosclerosis (hardening of the arteries) and the development of heart disease. Try sprinkling it with cinnamon rather than sugar to take away some of the tart taste.

**Mustard**

Try the hot, spicy kind you find in Asian import stores, specialty shops and exotic groceries. Dr. Jaya Henry of Oxford Polytechnic Institute in England, found that the amount of hot mustard normally called for in Mexican, Indian and Asian recipes, about one teaspoon, temporarily speeds up the metabolism, just as caffeine and the drug ephedrine do.

"But mustard is natural and totally safe," Henry says. "It can be used every day, and it really works. I was shocked to discover it can speed up the metabolism by as much as 20 to 25 percent for several hours." This can result in the body burning an extra 45 calories for every 700 consumed, Dr. Henry says.

**Peppers**

Hot, spicy chili peppers fall into the same category as hot mustard, Henry says. He studied them under the same circumstances as the mustard and they worked just as well. A mere three grams of chili peppers were added to a meal consisting of 766 total calories. The peppers' metabolism-raising properties worked like a charm, leading to what Henry call a diet-induced thermic effect. It doesn't take much to create the effect. Most salsa recipes call for four to eight chilies – that's not a lot.

Peppers are astonishingly rich in vitamins A and C, abundant in calcium, phosphorus, iron and magnesium, high in fiber, free of fat, low in sodium and have just 24 calories per cup.

**Potatoes**

We've got to be kidding, right? Wrong. Potatoes have developed the same "fattening" rap as bread, and it's unfair. Dr. John McDougal, director of the nutritional medicine clinic at St. Helena Hospital in Deer Park, California, says, "An excellent food with which to achieve rapid weight loss is the potato, at 0.6 calories per gram or about 85 calories per potato." A great source of fiber and potassium, they lower cholesterol and protect against strokes and heart disease.

Preparation and toppings are crucial. Steer clear of butter, milk and sour cream, or you'll blow it. Opt for yogurt instead.

**Rice**

An entire weight-loss plan, simple called the Rice Diet, was developed by Dr. William Kempner at Duke University in Durham, North Carolina. The diet, dating to the 1930's, makes rice the staple of your food intake. Later on, you gradually mix in various fruits and vegetables.

It produces stunning weight loss and medical results. The diet has been shown to reverse and cure kidney ailments and high blood pressure.

A cup of cooked rice (150 grams) contains about 178 calories – approximately one-third the number of calories found in an equivalent amount of beef or cheese. And remember, whole grain rice is much better for you than white rice.

**Soups**

Soup is good for you! Maybe not the canned varieties from the store – but old-fashioned, homemade soup promotes weight loss. A study by Dr. John Foreyt of Baylor College of Medicine in Houston, Texas, found that dieters who ate a bowl of soup before lunch and dinner lost more weight than dieters who didn't. In fact, the more soup they ate, the more weight they lost. And soup eaters tend to keep the weight off longer.

Naturally, the type of soup you eat makes a difference. Cream soups or those made of beef or pork are not your best bets. But here's a great recipe:

Slice three large onions, three carrots, four stalks of celery, one zucchini and one yellow squash. Place in a kettle. Add three cans crushed tomatoes, two packets low-sodium chicken bouillon, three cans water and one cup white wine (optional). Add tarragon, basil, oregano, and thyme and garlic powder. Boil, and then simmer for an hour. Serves six.

**Spinach**

Popeye really knew what he was talking about, according to Dr. Richard Shekelle, an epidemiologist at the University of Texas. Spinach has the ability to lower cholesterol, rev up the metabolism and burn away fat. Rich in iron, beta carotene and vitamins C and E, it supplies most of the nutrients you need.

**Tofu**

You just can't say enough about this health food from Asia. Also called soybean curd, it's basically tasteless, so any spice or flavoring you add blends with it nicely. A 2½" square has 86 calories and nine grams of protein. (Experts suggest an intake of about 40 grams per day.) Tofu contains calcium and iron, almost no sodium and not a bit of saturated fat. It makes your metabolism run on high and even lowers cholesterol. With different varieties available, the firmer tofus are goof for stir-frying or adding to soups and sauces while the softer ones are good for mashing, chopping and adding to salads.

**Potent Foods**

It would be unrealistic to think you could successfully lose weight and enjoy what you're eating with a mere handful of foods, no matter how delicious, nutritious and satisfying they may be. So we're going to add an extra roster of fat-fighting foods you can eat along with the great foods mentioned in the last section.

They'll lend different tastes and textures to every meal and provide a wide range of vitamins, minerals, proteins and other vital nutrients. Naturally, each one is high in fiber, low in fat and safe when it comes to sodium content, too.

Many have crunchiness and flavor we've come to desire in snack and nibbling foods. If you're like most of us, you may have a real junk food snacking habit – a habit you're going to have to change in order to slim down. Many of the foods in this section may be worthy substitutes.

**Barley**

This filling grain stacks up favorably to rice and potatoes. It has 170 calories per cooked cup, respectable levels of protein and fiber and relatively low fat. Roman gladiators ate this grain regularly for strength and actually complained when they had to eat meat.

Studies at the University of Wisconsin show that barley effectively lowers cholesterol by up to 15 percent and has powerful anti-cancer agents. Israeli scientists say it cures constipation better than laxatives - and that can promote weight loss, too.

Use it as a substitute for rice in salads, pilaf or stuffing, or add to soups and stews. You can also mix it with rice for an interesting texture. Ground into flour, it makes excellent breads and muffins.

**Beans**

Beans are one of the best sources of plant protein. Peas, beans and chickpeas are collectively known as legumes. Most common beans have 215 calories per cooked cup (lima beans go up to 260). They have the most protein with the least fat of any food, and they're high in potassium but low in sodium.

Plant protein is incomplete, which means that you need to add something to make it complete. Combine beans with a whole grain – rice, barley, wheat, corn – to provide the amino acids necessary to form a complete protein. Then you get the same top-quality protein as in meat with just a fraction of the fat.

Studies at the University of Kentucky and in the Netherlands show that eating beans regularly can lower cholesterol levels.

The most common complaint about beans is that they cause gas. Here's how to contain that problem, according to the U.S. Department of Agriculture (USDA): Before cooking, rinse the beans and remove foreign particles, put in a kettle and cover with boiling water, soak for four hours or longer, remove any beans that float to the top, and then cook the beans in fresh water.

**Berries**

This is the perfect weight-loss food. Berries have natural fructose sugar that satisfies your longing for sweets and enough fiber so you absorb fewer calories that you eat. British researchers found that the high content of insoluble fiber in fruits, vegetables and whole grains reduces the absorption of calories from foods enough to promote width loss without hampering nutrition.

Berries are a great source of potassium that can assist you in blood pressure control. Blackberries have 74 calories per cup, blueberries 81, raspberries 60 and strawberries 45. So use your imagination and enjoy the berry of your choice.

**Broccoli**

Broccoli is America's favorite vegetable, according to a recent poll. No wonder. A cup of cooked broccoli has a mere 44 calories. It delivers a staggering nutritional payload and is considered the number one cancer-fighting vegetable. It has no fat, loads of fiber, cancer fighting chemicals called indoles, carotene, 21 times the RDA of vitamin C and calcium.

When you're buying broccoli, pay attention to the color. The tiny florets should be rich green and free of yellowing. Stems should be firm.

## Buckwheat

It's great for pancakes, breads, cereal, and soups or alone as a grain dish commonly called kasha. It has 155 calories per cooked cup. Research at the All India Institute of Medical Sciences shows diets including buckwheat lead to excellent blood sugar regulation, resistance to diabetes and lowered cholesterol levels. You cook buckwheat the same way you would rice or barley. Bring two to three cups of water to a boil, add the grain, cover the pan, turn down the heat and simmer for 20 minutes or until the water is absorbed.

## Cabbage

This Eastern Europe staple is a true wonder food. There are only 33 calories in a cup of cooked shredded cabbage, and it retains all its nutritional goodness no matter how long you cook it. Eating cabbage raw (18 calories per shredded cup), cooked, as sauerkraut (27 calories per drained cup) or coleslaw (calories depend on dressing) only once a week is enough to protect against colon cancer. And it may be a longevity-enhancing food. Surveys in the United States, Greece and Japan show that people who eat a lot of it have the least colon cancer and the lowest death rates overall.

## Carrots

What list of health-promoting, fat-fighting foods would be complete without Bugs Bunny's favorite? A medium-sized carrot carries about 55 calories and is a nutritional powerhouse. The orange color comes from beta carotene, a powerful cancer-preventing nutrient (provitamin A).

Chop and toss them with pasta, grate them into rice or add them to a stir-fry. Combine them with parsnips, oranges, raisins, lemon juice, chicken, potatoes, broccoli or lamb to create flavorful dishes. Spice them with tarragon, dill, cinnamon or nutmeg. Add finely chopped carrots to soups and spaghetti sauce – they impart a natural sweetness without adding sugar.

## Chicken

White meat contains 245 calories per four ounce serving and dark meat, 285. It's an excellent source of protein, iron, niacin and zinc. Skinned chicken is healthiest, but most experts recommend waiting until after cooking to remove it because the skin keeps the meat moist during cooking.

## Corn

It's really a grain – not a vegetable – and is another food that's gotten a bum rap. People think it has little to offer nutritionally and that just isn't so. There are 178 calories in a cup of cooked kernels. It contains good amounts of iron, zinc and potassium, and University of Nebraska researchers say it delivers a high-quality of protein, too.

The Tarahumara Indians of Mexico eat corn, beans and hardly anything else. Virgil Brown, M.D., of Mount Sinai School of

Medicine in New York, points out that high blood cholesterol and cardiovascular heart disease are almost nonexistent among them.

**Cottage Cheese**

As long as we're talking about losing weight and fat-fighting foods, we had to mention cottage cheese.

Low-fat (2%) cottage cheese has 205 calories per cup and is admirably low in fat, while providing respectable amounts of calcium and the B vitamin riboflavin. Season with spices such a dill, or garden fresh vegetable such a scallions and chives for extra zip.

To make it sweeter, add raisins or one of the fruit spreads with no sugar added. You can also use cottage cheese in cooking, baking, fillings and dips where you would otherwise use sour cream or cream cheese.

**Figs**

Fiber-rich figs are low in calories at 37 per medium (2.25" diameter) raw fig and 48 per dried fig. A recent study by the USDA demonstrated that they contribute to a feeling of fullness and prevent overeating. Subjects actually complained of being asked to eat too much food when fed a diet containing more figs than a similar diet with an identical number of calories.

Serve them with other fruits and cheeses. Or poach them in fruit juice and serve them warm or cold. You can stuff them with mild white cheese or puree them to use as a filling for cookies and low-calorie pastries.

**Fish**

The health benefits of fish are greater than experts imagined – and they've always considered it a health food.

The calorie count in the average four-ounce serving of a deep-sea fish runs from a low of 90 calories in abalone to a high of 236 in herring. Water-packed tuna, for example, has 154 calories. It's hard to gain weight eating seafood.

As far back as 1985, articles in the New England Journal of Medicine showed a clear link between eating fish regularly and lower rates of heart disease. The reason is that oils in fish thin the blood, reduce blood pressure and lower cholesterol.

Dr. Joel Kremer, at Albany Medical College in New York, discovered that daily supplements of fish oil brought dramatic relief to the inflammation and stiff joints of rheumatoid arthritis.

**Greens**

We're talking collard, chicory, beet, kale, mustard, Swiss chard and turnip greens. They all belong to the same family as spinach, and that's one of the super-stars. No matter how hard you try, you can't load a cup of plain cooked greens with any more than 50 calories.

They're full of fiber, loaded with vitamins A and C, and free of fat. You can use them in salads, soups, casseroles or any dish where you would normally use spinach.

**Kiwi**

This New Zealand native is a sweet treat at only 46 calories per fruit. Chinese public health officials praise the tasty fruit for its high vitamin C content and potassium. It stores easily in the refrigerator for up to a month. Most people like it peeled, but the fuzzy skin is also edible.

**Leeks**

These members of the onion family look like giant scallions, and are every bit as healthful and flavorful as their better-known cousins. They come as close to calorie-free as it gets at a mere 32 calories per cooked cup.

You can poach or broil halved leeks and then marinate them in vinaigrette or season with Romano cheese, fine mustard or herbs. They also make a good soup.

**Lettuce**

People think lettuce is nutritionally worthless, but nothing could be farther from the truth. You can't leave it out of your weight-loss plans, not at 10 calories per cup of raw romaine. It provides a lot of filling bulk for so few calories. And it's full of vitamin C, too. Go beyond iceberg lettuce with Boston, bibb and cos varieties or try watercress, arugula, radicchio, dandelion greens, purslane and even parsley to liven up your salads.

**Melons**

Now, here's great taste and great nutrition in a low-calorie package! One cup of cantaloupe balls has 62 calories, on cup of casaba balls has 44 calories, one cup of honeydew balls has 62 calories and one cup of watermelon balls has 49 calories. They have some of the highest fiber content of any food and are delicious. Throw in handsome quantities of vitamins A and C plus a whopping 547 mgs of potassium in that cup of cantaloupe, and you have a fat-burning health food beyond compare.

## Oats

A cup of oatmeal or oat bran has only 110 calories. And oats help you lose weight. Subjects in Dr. James Anderson's landmark 12-year study at the University of Kentucky lost three pounds in two months simply by adding 100 grams (3.5 ounces) of oat bran to their daily food intake and nothing else. Just don't expect oats alone to perform miracles – you have to eat a balanced diet for total health.

## Onions

Flavorful, aromatic, inexpensive and low in calories, onions deserve a regular place in your diet. One cup of chopped raw onions has only 60 calories, and one raw medium onion (2.15" diameter) has just 42.

They control cholesterol, thin the blood, protect against cholesterol and may have some value in counteracting allergic reactions. Most of all, onions taste good and they're good for you.

Partially boil, peel and bake, basting with olive oil and lemon juice. Or sauté them in white wine and basil, then spread over pizza. Or roast them in sherry and serve over paste.

**Pasta**

The Italians had it right all along. A cup of cooked paste (without a heavy sauce) has only 155 calories and fits the description of a perfect starch-centered staple. Analysis at the American

Institute of Baking shows pasta is rich in six minerals, including manganese, iron, phosphorus, copper, magnesium and zinc. Also be sure to consider whole wheat pastas, which are even healthier.

**Sweet Potatoes**

You can make a meal out of them and not worry about gaining a pound – and you sure won't walk away from the table feeling hungry. Each sweet potato has about 103 calories. Their creamy orange flesh is one of the best sources of vitamin A you can consume.

You can bake steam or microwave them. Or add them to casseroles, soups and many other dishes. Flavor with lemon juice or vegetable broth instead of butter.

**Tomatoes**

A medium tomato (2.5" diameter) has only about 25 calories. These garden delights are low in fat and sodium, high in potassium and rich in fiber.

A survey at Harvard Medical School found that the chances of dying of cancer are lowest among people who eat tomatoes (or strawberries) every week.

And don't overlook canned crushed, peeled, whole or stewed tomatoes. They make sauces, casseroles and soups taste great while retaining their nutritional goodness and low-calorie status. Even plain old spaghetti sauce is a fat-burning bargain when served over pasta, so think about introducing tomatoes into your diet

**Turkey**

Give thanks to those pilgrims for starting the wonderful tradition of Thanksgiving turkey. It just so happens that this health food disguised as meat is good year-round for weight control.

A four-ounce serving of roasted white meat turkey has 177 calories and dark meat has 211.

Sadly, many folks are still unaware of the versatility and flavor of ground turkey. Anything hamburger can do, ground turkey can do at least as well, from conventional burgers to spaghetti sauce to meat loaf.

Some ground turkey contains skin which slightly increases the fat content. If you want to keep it really lean, opt for ground breast meat. But since this has no added fat, you'll need to add filler to make burgers or meat loaf hold together.

Four ounces of ground turkey has approximately 170 calories and nine grams of fat – about what you'd find in 2.5 teaspoons of butter or margarine. Incredibly, the same amount of regular ground beef (21% fat) has 298 calories and 23 grams of fat.

Buying turkey has become easy. It's no longer necessary to buy a whole bird unless you want to. Ground turkey is available fresh or frozen, as are individual parts of the bird, including drumsticks, thighs, breasts and cutlets.

**Yogurt**

The non-fat variety of plain yogurt has 120 calories per cup and low-fat, 144. It delivers a lot of protein and, like any dairy food, is rich in calcium and contains zinc and riboflavin.

Yogurt is handy as a breakfast food – cut a banana into it and add the cereal of your choice.

You can find ways to use it in other types of cooking, to – sauces, soups, dips, toppings, stuffing and spreads. Many kitchen gadget departments even sell a simple funnel for making yogurt cheese.

Yogurt can replace heavy creams and whole milk in a wide range of dishes, saving scads of fat and calories.

You can substitute half or all of the higher fat ingredients. Be creative. For example, combine yogurt, garlic powder, lemon juice, and a dash of pepper and Worcestershire sauce and use it to top a baked potato instead of piling on fat-laden sour cream.

Supermarkets and health food stores sell a variety of yogurts, many with added fruit and sugar. To control calories and fat content, buy plain non-fat yogurt and add fruit yourself. Apple butter or fruit spreads with little or no added sugar are an excellent way to turn plain yogurt into a delectable sweet treat.

# About the Author

Janet Simpson was overweight during her early teens. She had difficulties controlling her food intake. Both of her parents are suffering from diabetes as well. During college, Janet realized that if she will not act soon, she will end up having the same health problems as her parent which she doesn't like.

Janet then devoted her time to read books, attended different gym class and underwent many meal plans but unfortunately nothing seemed to work for her. She then created a formula of her own which is just perfect for her. This prompted Janet to write to be an inspiration to all.

www.ingramcontent.com/pod-product-compliance
Lightning Source LLC
Chambersburg PA
CBHW070044260726
48658CB00002B/718